GW00544707

BREAST DISEASE

IS THE MAIN CAUSE OF BREAST DISEASE STARING US IN THE FACE?

ANTOINETTE CLANCY

ON STREAM

Published 1997 for A. Clancy in by On Stream Publications Ltd., Cloghroe, Blarney, Co. Cork Ireland.

© A. Clancy

Tel/fax: + 353 21 385798. e-mail address: onstream@indigo.ie

A CIP record for this book is available from the British Library.

Printed in Ireland by Colour Books

The moral right of the author has been asserted.

All rights reserved. No part of this publication may be reproduced in any form or by any means, electronic or mechanical, including photography, recording or any information storage or retrieval system, without permission in writing from the publisher, except for review purposes. This book is sold subject to the condition that it shall not, by way of trade or otherwise, be lent, re-sold or otherwise circulated without the publisher's prior consent, in any form of binding or cover other than that in which it is published and without similar condition, including this condition, being imposed on the subsequent purchaser.

ISBN: 1 897685 84 X

TO MARTIN

WITH LOVE

Introduction

Gone are the days when there was enough animal life lurking in a head of lettuce to provide material for a television wildlife programme. It used to take a little time and care to clean your greens if you didn't want to end up with a slug in your salad. Or worse still - half a slug. All that has changed.

Today we can go to the supermarket and buy a perfectly shaped, wildlife-free lettuce, grown on chemically-treated land and wrapped in chemically-made see-through plastic film.

We are no longer willing to accept food containing a harmless creepy-crawly which can be removed, but we are quite happy to eat the same food when it has been laced with drugs or adulterated with chemicals. If we are told that our food is "perfectly safe", we accept this without question, and, as long as it looks OK, think no more about it. It is only when media headlines tell a different story that most people start to question what they are eating. Once the story is out of the news we forget all about it.

We are going through a time when our water, food, land and air can contain extremely expensive chemicals so that we can have cheaper food which lasts longer, and looks enticing.

These goals are achieved, but what do we know of the cost?

This book tells my own story: how I have learned to count the cost through my own experience of breast disease, and my search to find the cause.

DISCOVERY

Despite all the fantastic medical advancements of this century, such as the discovery of antibiotics, immunisation and genetic engineering, for women there is still the nightmare of breast cancer. If we were to believe all the media hype about apparent "miracle breakthroughs," one might be forgiven for believing that women didn't die of breast cancer any more. One might even assume that all we have to do is to look routinely for signs of the deadly disease and that, by going through this ritual, we may find a lump at a stage where we can be cured before it is too late.

The trauma of discovering a breast lump can only be understood if it has been experienced. I was in my early twenties and my two children were just tots when I discovered my first breast lump. There were weeks of hell waiting for a bed in hospital, and then more distressing suspense awaiting the results of the biopsy - a test which finally showed the lump to be harmless. The relief was enormous, and the knowledge that there was still a life ahead of me with my children was the best news ever.

Some months later, I discovered another lump and went through the whole ordeal all over again.

When I next found a large lump in one breast and a small one in the other, it nearly sent me berserk. It began to look as though my whole existence would consist of going in and out of hospitals and living in fear. I didn't *want* to examine my breasts regularly to look for signs of possible cancer. I just wanted to know *why* these so-called "harmless" lumps appeared, what caused them and why some women got them while others didn't.

Would the lumps go away if I did nothing? There was only one way to find out and, saying nothing to anyone, I started doing some research of my own into benign breast disease. But at the end of a year I was no wiser.

Let me stress that I am not for one moment suggesting that women simply ignore a breast lump, or that they follow my example during the following years. This book is *not* about treatment of breast cancer, but looks at possible *causes* for the increase of the disease during the past thirty to forty years.

Ten years later, in my early thirties, I noticed that a mole which had been on my arm throughout my life had begun to change. It was now three times the size, irregular in shape, had changed colour and was red around the edges. It was growing rapidly, and the changes in size could be seen from week to week. I knew enough about skin cancer to know that it was no longer a harmless mole. And so it occurred to me that the lump in my breast might be cancerous and that the change in the mole was due to secondaries. If this was the case, then there was no one to blame but myself. What had I done?

That night was passed lying awake remembering a childhood spent playing on the beach across the road from our house. My friends and I used to be able to peel off layers of skin only a few days after we had been sunburned. We had never used any type of protection cream - I don't remember there being any such thing when I was a child. I remembered the years that I had lived in Africa, with its long daylight hours of sunshine. I had done all the things that we are advised today not to do. But so had all my friends who grew up on the same road as me, and none of them had died of skin cancer as far as I knew. It seemed to me that there must be something else which was causing the change in the mole on my arm. Maybe that was what I wanted to believe.

Experts keep telling us that even one episode of sunburn in childhood is enough to cause skin cancer later on. But how do they know? Where did they find sufficiently large numbers of people who never got sunburned in their lives to compare with those who did get sunburned? I don't know of many adults who never got sunburned to some extent at some point in their lives. If skin cancer is caused by the sun's rays acting together with something else, and it is not yet known what the "something else" is, then it is reasonable to warn people not to get sunburned.

Perhaps it was my diet: all the chemicals which are sprayed on food and indeed, all the chemicals which are put into it, such as flavourings, colourings and preservatives. But, surely, I had been eating the very same foods for years on end, chemicals and all.

A doctor friend examined the mole and told me not to worry, that he would get a surgeon to see me straight away. He nearly had a fit when I told him that I was not sure about having surgery. After all, it seemed to me that once the mole was removed, then there was no way of knowing whether or not changes in diet and lifestyle would have had any effect on it. Of course, without treatment I might not be alive to find out anything one way or the other.

As there had not been even a slight change in the mole the previous summer, I felt it must have been due to some alteration in my lifestyle during the previous few years. I had lived abroad for fifteen years, and had only been back in Ireland for a year at the time, but could not see how that would have made any difference. And then it slowly dawned on me.

I had been on Hormone Replacement Therapy (HRT), in the form of oestrogen only, for a little over a year, as treatment for the menopause. I decided to stop taking the drug to see if it made any difference to the mole.

A few weeks after that, a surgeon friend noticed the mole. I told him what I was trying out with regard to abandoning my HRT. He told me in no uncertain terms that it was obviously a malignant melanoma, and that without immediate treatment I would be dead in six months. He showed me a colour picture of a malignant melanoma in a medical book, and it looked exactly the same as the mole on my arm.

It was a worrying situation, but I really believed that there must have been something apart from the sun's rays which was causing this condition. I decided to cover the mole with medical tape, which acts like a second skin and didn't have to be removed for bathing, left it undisturbed, and wrote a note in my diary to examine it again in a year's time. The tape acted as a camouflage and prevented me from seeing the mole. I was afraid of my resolve weakening if I could see it growing, and of being tempted to have it removed. What was certain was that cells inside the mole were changing and multiplying rapidly. At times, I was petrified by my decision to ignore medical advice, and at one point I made an appointment with my GP to have it seen to, but cancelled before the consultation.

Eventually the whole business stopped being uppermost in my mind and the day finally came to remove the tape.

The mole had reverted to its original size, colour and shape. This meant that the cells had stopped multiplying, and that some had died off, as could be seen by the size reduction. I couldn't believe my eyes.

The fact that the mole had reverted back to its original form could have been due to stopping the HRT, to covering the mole, or to something else altogether. The fact that it had changed in the first place may very well have been due to having been sunburnt umpteen times as a child, and then taking hormones later on. After all, to continuously burn one's skin does damage it, and changes in hormone levels also affect the skin. (For example, a woman's nipples change colour during pregnancy. Also, the earlier contraceptive pill, which contained higher doses of oestrogen than in the Pill today, caused dark patches on the skin of some women who took it.) The following summer, I went out in the sun as usual, leaving the mole uncovered, and yet there were no changes to it.

This demonstrated, to myself at least, that my mole was oestrogen-dependent, in that, when the artificial oestrogens were stopped (discontinuing HRT), the mole reverted to being harmless. It would be most unwise for others to assume that the same thing was likely to be true of a mole of theirs which showed signs of change. Under such circumstances they must seek medical advice.

The point of my story is not that you should ignore changes in a mole, but rather that if you do have one or more harmless moles, perhaps you should think twice before agreeing to take additional hormones (particularly oestrogens), as they could cause cancerous changes, and you might not be as lucky as I was.

I then started to research Hormone Replacement Therapy (HRT). Some scientific papers proved that it was "God's gift to women" while others proved the opposite. There was no mention of an increased risk of skin cancers in patients who took oestrogens.

It was 1975, my research was getting nowhere, and so I once again decided to leave it to the scientists. But, despite what the experts told me about the danger of developing osteoporosis (brittle bone disease), I was not going to take HRT.

It was certainly true that on first taking this hormone (oestrogen), there were no more hot flushes or night sweats, nor did I feel like blowing my top if someone so much as left a door open. There were, however, headaches and painful breasts, which I was told were "just the side effects of HRT". As soon as I came off the hormone treatment, all the symptoms of the menopause returned, and the side-effects of the HRT became less. But, as time passed, my body seemed to adjust itself. The symptoms of the menopause disappeared and the mole wasn't causing any more trouble. I checked my breasts and found that there was no sign of a lump.

There is now scientific evidence to show that taking oestrogen, whether in the form of the Pill or in HRT, increases the risk of malignant melanoma.

BREAST PAIN

All went well until 1981, when I began once more to suffer very painful breasts. This time, it could not have been due to the side effects of HRT, as I wasn't on any form of hormone treatment.

Many women get slight pain and/or discomfort before a period, and that is normal. But this pain was present most of the time, and was so severe that it prevented me from sleeping properly. My breasts were so agonisingly sensitive that even a hug from one of my children would have me yelping with pain.

I asked a few of my friends if they had ever experienced this type of breast pain and one of them had. She told me that her doctor had diagnosed it as normal. Normal! As far as I was concerned, this degree of pain was nature's way of letting me know that something was wrong, and this time I was determined to find the cause.

Earlier this century, women who complained of severe breast pain were not taken seriously by the "experts". They were looked upon as frustrated, unhappy women who hadn't had a child. In 1938, Dr. Hedley Atkins wrote: *"My own impression of many of these patients is the same as that of Sir Astley Cooper, that they are of an irritable and suggestive nature."*

This was the view held by the medical profession in general, and continued to be so for decades. It was not until the late 1970s that some doctors proved that Dr. Atkins, Sir Astley Cooper and their colleagues were incorrect. This won't come as any surprise to women with severe breast pain.

The medical term for breast pain is *mastalgia*. It is defined as severe pain felt mainly in the upper, outer part of the breasts (near the arms) which become tender to the touch. The breasts can feel lumpy. All symptoms get worse before a period, or during an equivalent part of the cycle in women who no longer get periods. In certain cases, the symptoms persist for such a long time each month that some women are in constant pain. Mastalgia is fairly rare in women who have been through the menopause, unless they are on HRT.

According to one scientific paper, mastalgia was caused by a high intake of caffeine. I gave up all food and drinks containing caffeine for five months and had no relief from the pain.

I tried Evening Primrose Oil as directed but it made no difference.

Progesterone treatment, which was shown to bring some relief to women with mastalgia, gave me lower abdominal pain, and made no difference to the breast pain.

Finally I was given Tamoxifen, which is an anti-oestrogen drug. This worked. After a few weeks treatment, I was pain-free.

It was indeed a great relief to be free of pain but the reasoning behind the treatment made no sense to me. Here was I, a post-menopausal woman who had been advised to take oestrogen to prevent my bones from falling to bits because my own body wasn't producing enough of the hormone to keep them in one piece, now needing a drug which blocked the effect of the little natural oestrogen that my body *did* manage to produce!

I gave up taking Tamoxifen and the breast pain subsequently returned, persisting almost constantly for months. Then, out of the blue, the pain got better, in spite of the fact that I hadn't taken any form of treatment.

The only change in my life at the time was the departure of my eldest son to London to take up a new job. I was sad to see him leave home, and, had I been experiencing the pain at that time, it might well have been put down to the start of the "empty nest" syndrome. However, I was quite looking forward to having an empty nest. Perhaps Sir Astley Cooper was right about women: *"It's all in their minds"*.

There was one other very small change after my son left home. He loved eating chicken, so we would have it once a week. After he left we changed to eating fish instead. The breast pain disappeared.

I began to wonder if chicken could cause mastalgia. After all, poultry was legally being fed hormones (including oestrogens) as growth promoters.

I returned to eating chicken once a week, and within three weeks the breast pain was back.

During the following eight years, I gave up eating all meat, except for the purpose of testing the effects of eating or not eating meat on my breast pain.

Beef and lamb didn't cause any problems, but each time I ate even three ounces of chicken the pain returned and continued for weeks.

Organic poultry is hard to get, but a friend gave me some chickens from her own registered organic farm. I divided these into measured portions, kept them in the freezer, and started doing trials on myself once more.

I did *not* get mastalgia while eating organic chicken, despite eating it up to three times each week for months.

This now proved, in my own case, that eating ordinary (non-organic) chicken caused me to get mastalgia.

Questions

The questions to be answered now were:

* Why should ordinary chicken cause me to have mastalgia?

* Did it cause mastalgia in other women?

* Was there any connection between mastalgia and breast cancer?

At this stage I knew that:

* When I was taking oestrogens in the form of HRT I got mastalgia.

* When I ate chicken which had been fed oestrogen I got mastalgia.

* When I ate organic poultry, or adopted a poultry-free diet I remained free from pain.

I spent months on end, over a period of years, taking courses in Epidemiology, which is the study of how diseases occur in various groups of people. Part of the courses included conducting surveys, and this was far more difficult than I had ever imagined.

My free time was spent reading surveys and clinical trials on breast disease, the effects of the Pill, HRT and anything else which might shed some light on breast disease and its possible causes.

Eventually, in 1992, I started work on my own survey to find out what percentage of women had mastalgia, and whether or not there was any connection between mastalgia and meat-eating, taking the Pill, having HRT or smoking. This type of survey had never been carried out before.

Considering that millions of people eat meat which is produced using of an assortment of growth-promoting hormones, there is an extraordinary lack of scientific research on the effects of these hormones on food.

After months of work, my first survey had to be scrapped as the return rate was too low. Out of every 100 questionnaires received by women, only eight were returned fully answered. Some were, of course, not returned at all, but that is to be expected. With such a low return rate, the results would not prove anything one way or the other, as there was a possibility that the women who returned the forms were mainly those who suffered from mastalgia.

There was nothing for it but to go walking from house to house. I wanted to talk to the women myself, and prayed that they would be willing to answer the 25 questions in my questionnaire. They were extremely co-operative, and the numbers taking part were far higher than would normally be expected in this type of survey.

The information was collected, put into the computer and sent away for analysis.

Results

My survey showed that roughly 22% of women had mastalgia. However, an even more important finding was that those women who ate more that six ounces of ordinary (non-organic) chicken each week were over four times more likely to get mastalgia than those who ate less than this amount.

Nine out of ten individual women in the survey who went to their GP with severe breast pain had been told that such pain was normal, and only one of the women surveyed was offered treatment.

If women go to their doctor with severe breast pain and are told that such pain is normal, they tend not to return. This leads to a situation where women believe that severe breast pain is normal, and where doctors believe that all a woman needs for "what she calls" severe breast pain is reassurance that the pain is not due to cancer.

TESTING THE RESULTS

To test the results of my survey, nine women who had experienced severe mastalgia for a minimum of one year and who were not on the Pill or HRT were asked to give up eating all forms of poultry. They were not told why they were being asked to do this, and they believed that other women were being asked to give up beef and other meats. Six weeks later, eight of these women were completely free of pain.

They were then asked to continue eating chicken as before, but four of the women were so pleased to be free of pain for the first time in years that they were not willing to resume. The remaining four women did start to eat chicken again, and their pain returned in two to three weeks. All nine women were checked over a period of ten months. At the end of this time, eight of the nine women were able to remain pain-free by excluding poultry from their diet, or by reducing the amount of poultry eaten. The ninth woman in the trial was advised at an early stage to return to her doctor.

When I had breast pain in the early eighties, it was perfectly legal to use hormones as growth promoters. However, it is worth noting that in 1988 Ireland brought in regulations banning the use of all hormones in farm animals for human consumption. *Yet there are no routine hormone tests for these substances carried out on poultry.* On numerous occasions over a period of two years, such tests were requested and not one could be performed in the entire country.

I attempted to conduct a second survey to compare women who ate only registered organic meat or were vegetarians with women who ate ordinary meat. As it was only possible to contact seventeen women who did not eat ordinary meat, I did not continue with this line of enquiry. However, of these seventeen women I spoke to, sixteen never had mastalgia, and the remaining woman only had it for a few months during the previous few years. During that time she had not eaten meat, but had changed from eating a very varied vegetarian diet to one which contained high levels of soya. When she changed back to her normal, much more varied vegetarian diet, her breast pain got better and she has remained pain-free ever since.

Soya contains very high levels of natural oestrogens which may have caused her problem. The full results of this survey and clinical trial are at the back of this book.

THE FACTS

Despite what we are being told, breast cancer has increased by almost 50% during the past 40 years and continues to increase slightly each year. This continued slight increase may be due to increased diagnoses of the disease.

The proportion of women with breast cancer who die from the disease is as high as ever. The cause is still unknown.

Diet is thought to be the most important *single* factor in the cause of breast cancer. As we cannot give up eating, it is necessary to find out which item or items in our diet (or lacking in our diet) may cause the disease.

Breast cancer rates are highest in Western countries where diet is high in meat and fat.

In Eastern countries where the diet is semi-vegetarian, breast cancer rates are low.

Migrants from Eastern countries who go to the USA quickly change to a Western diet, and their breast cancer rates rise correspondingly within 20 years. This would seem to indicate that the cause is due to diet or environment.

Vegetarian women are 40% less likely to get breast cancer than women who eat meat.

Women who are overweight have an increased risk of breast cancer. Oestrogen is stored in fat cells, and so, the more fat cells we have, the more oestrogen we can store in our bodies.

Higher than normal levels of oestrogen in the body increase the risk of breast cancer.

Women who suffer from benign breast disease such as lumps, cysts or severe pain in the breast which is not cancer, have an increased risk of getting cancer later on.

Roughly 8% of breast cancers are hereditary. This means that a small number of women may inherit a gene which makes them more prone to getting cancer. Put another way, 92% of breast cancers are not hereditary.

Most breast cancers belong to the group of cancers which are hormone-dependent. This means that the cancer needs oestrogen to grow. Castration of women, by removing their ovaries to reduce their own production of hormones, was part of the treatment until drugs which cause a medical castration were found.

Long-term use of the contraceptive pill increases the risk of breast cancer.

There is a significantly increased risk of breast cancer among women who have a long-term use of HRT.

One of the side effects of the IVF (In Vitro Fertilization) programme, where women are put on hormones to produce eggs for fertilization, is an increased risk of breast and ovarian cancer.

Radiation, chemicals and viruses have been proven to cause cancer in humans.

Hundreds of chemicals are known to cause cancer in animals

In the canine world, bitches who are spayed are 35% less likely to get cancer than those who are not spayed. As dogs do not normally take the Pill or HRT, could the common denominator between their diet and that of women be the consumption of meat and fat?

Women who get early menopause are less likely to get breast cancer, and those who have a late menopause are more likely to get the disease. Indeed, women who have their ovaries surgically removed before the age of 35 have significantly less risk of developing breast cancer than women who go on to have a natural menopause.

It looks as though the longer we produce our own natural oestrogens, the higher our chances are of getting breast cancer. If this is so, it does not seem like a good idea to take extra oestrogens in the form of HRT.

*

Women were having the menopause at the same age 50 years ago, when the rate of breast cancer was far lower than it is now.

Could it be that we are consuming more oestrogens or oestrogen-like substances today than we were fifty years ago?

Poultry consumption has increased 100% during the past twenty years, and this has further increased since the BSE scare.

Some experts tell us that women did not live long enough a hundred years ago to even reach the menopause. This is not true. Life expectancy was then about 45 years, but that does not mean that people only lived to be 45. What brought down the average life span at the time was the high death rate among children. For example, if one hundred people born in Timbuktu all lived to be 70, their average life span would be 70. However, if 50 of these people died before the age of two, and the remainder lived to be 70, then the average life span for those people would be about 35 years. One hundred years ago, females who managed to survive childhood went on to live to be 65 or more - long past the age of menopause.

SEARCHING FOR CANCER

Breast cancer is extremely rare in women under the age of 35. It is true that it is the most common cause of death in women between the age of 35 and 55, but it must be remembered that the number of deaths among women due to *any* cause in this age group is low. However, one third of women who die from breast cancer do so before the age of 65.

As there is no known way to prevent breast cancer, we are advised to look for signs of the disease by examining our breasts regularly. This constant emphasis on early diagnosis of breast cancer by self-examination of the breasts causes widespread fear among women. Yet we are continually advised to do so, even though early detection of small cancerous lumps by this method seems to have little if any effect on the outcome. Most women do not routinely examine their breasts. This is not surprising as, consciously or unconsciously, they do not want to spend their lives looking for signs of a disease which may cause their death.

The outcome of screening for breast cancer is that many cancers are detected earlier than might otherwise be expected. Apparent extra time survived after diagnosis is referred to as "lead time."

For example, a woman whom I shall call "Mary" examined her breasts every month and found a tiny lump when she was 55 which turned out to be cancerous. She had surgery, medical treatment and routine check-ups. It took years for her to come to terms with the fact that she had cancer. Even then, every time she wasn't feeling well she thought the cancer had come back, but she lived to be 72 years of age.

"Ann", on the other hand, didn't bother to examine her breasts and went on her merry way until she was 68, when she then noticed a lump in her breast. She also had surgery and medical treatment and died four years later, aged 72.

Mary and Ann may have had cancers that were identical in type and had started to grow at the same time, in which case both women survived the cancer for the same duration. However, Mary had 17 years of worry, while Ann had only four years. Mary's cancer was diagnosed sooner than Ann's, so it looks as if Mary survived cancer longer than Ann.

If there were a group of "Marys", they would be described as having a 100%, 5-year survival rate, and 100% 10-year survival rate. Indeed, these Marys could also come under the heading of 100% cure rate. On the other hand, a group of Anns would be described as having a zero 5-year survival rate or, put another way, a 100% death rate within 5 years.

These conclusions are perfectly true. However, we take it for granted that Mary *benefited* from early diagnosis. But in this hypothetical case both women died at the age of 72 from the same condition.

We know Mary's cancer was just barely detectable at the age of 55, 17 years before she died. Is it not possible that the same was true for Ann's cancer, except for the fact that she didn't know about it until four years before she also died?

MAMMOGRAPHY

As well as self-examination, we are also encouraged to have mammography screening. This is an X-Ray scan which will show up any signs of cancer at an even earlier stage than breast examination by hand.

There has been no significant reduction in deaths from breast cancer since mammography programmes were introduced.

Roughly 5% of mammograms turn out to be positive. Had I been one of the 5%, I might feel lucky to have found the cancer at such an early stage. However, it has also been shown that of the 5% which show up positive, roughly 90% of these are false positives. These patients do not have cancer at all. This would only have been discovered after they had been through unnecessary fear and a biopsy (the taking of a tissue sample). They may even have had a mastectomy "just to be on the safe side."

Worse still is the number of false negative results which occur with the use of mammography. About 12% of screened women are given a false negative result, which means that they are reassured that they are fine, when, in fact, they have cancer.

In 1990, Professor Michael Baum, who is an international expert on breast cancer, helped to set up the first national screening programme in Britain. He has now said (in 1995) that such screenings should be scrapped, because "they are not worth doing." He resigned from the NHS breast cancer advisory group.

It is beneficial to have a cancer removed before it spreads, but to what lengths we must go to find out whether or not we have the disease is a question which needs serious thought.

Is it reasonable to constantly worry the entire female population into becoming part of one huge clinical trial? If all the measures taken at present have done little to reduce death rates from breast cancer, will the next step be to remove women's breasts before there are any signs of the disease whatsoever? This would certainly reduce the rates of breast cancer.

Many women have had their breasts removed because of their fear of cancer, and not because they have actually had it. Some have had a mastectomy without even having had a test which would show whether or not they had the gene which would make them more prone to getting cancer, even though the test was available. It must also be pointed out that breast cancer does *not* develop in most women with a family history of the disease.

*

The following is a true story.

"Jane Smith" examined her breasts regularly and found a lump. She had a biopsy and it was found to be harmless. Over the next few years, she found more lumps. Each time she found a lump, she underwent a biopsy and was told she was fine. She was finally told to ignore her breast lumps. This she tried to do, but when she discovered yet another, she was again worried out of her mind. Her doctor examined her and told her it wasn't cancer. For years, she had been told that she must look for lumps in her breasts and have each lump examined, and now she was being told she didn't need to have this done. If her doctors couldn't tell beforehand whether or not each lump was cancerous, how could they know now?

She wanted another biopsy done to put her mind at ease. She was told she had cancer phobia. Perhaps this was true, but she got her phobia from listening to the experts. Finally, in desperation, she had both breasts removed, as it was the only way that she felt she could cope with her problem. She did not have a family history of breast cancer, but she had breasts, and without them she knew she couldn't get breast cancer.

Thousands of healthy women have had their breasts removed because of their fear of cancer.

CURE?

There is no cure for many diseases such as diabetes, but, with treatment, people can live normal lives. We do not expect to hear that a person is cured of diabetes. On the other hand, TB can be cured. Patients are given treatment which kills the germ, and they can then expect to live out the remainder of their lives without the disease and without treatment.

When we hear that a person has been cured of cancer, most people believe that the cancer cells have similarly been killed off, and that those who have had the disease will then live out the remainder of their lives without it. They are cured. Wrong.

When it comes to cancer, the medical profession distort the word "cure". When they use this word, they often refer to women who have improved, or to those who live for five years after diagnosis. The patient might die the following month, but they still come under the heading of being "cured." Why are we being misled?

Cancer does recur in many women after surgery and medical treatment, but with further treatment some can live on into old age. It is also interesting to note that women diagnosed with early breast cancer who refused all treatment have done as well as many of those who have been treated. This only goes to show that the progression of breast cancer still remains a mystery.

PREVENTION

Many cancers can be prevented once the cancer-causing agents are discovered.

In the past, skin cancer killed many people who worked in the coal-tar industries. Those who inhaled fumes from the coal-tar were associated with high rates of lung cancer.

While asbestos was being widely used in industry, the incidence of lung cancer among workers was ten times higher than normal.

Chemicals in the manufacture of dyes were linked to the high incidence of bladder cancer among workers. Women working in tableware factories put into their mouths the small paint brush they were using (which had been dipped in these dyes) in order to give it the fine point necessary for the work they were doing. This caused them to ingest chemicals which caused the increase in bladder cancer.

Certain pesticides were removed from the market when they were found to cause cancer in animals, and when they were also found in food sprayed with those pesticides.

Once the cause of these cancers was discovered and removed, cancer rates dropped dramatically.

Cancer of the lung used to be a relatively rare condition. However, a major increase in cigarette smoking took place early this century, and in countries where smoking was popular, deaths from lung cancer rose alarmingly. It was not until 1950 that medical evidence began to link cigarette smoking with lung cancer. At that time, Doctors Doll and Hill wrote a paper which showed that smoking was a major cause of lung cancer, and that the rate of this disease increased in proportion to the number of cigarettes smoked.

Like many before them who had come up with a new idea, they were ridiculed by their colleagues. With hindsight it seems that the cause was staring us in the face.

Another factor contributing to the high lung cancer rate this century is air pollution due to industrial and car emissions. City residents who are non-smokers have a 15% higher incidence of lung cancer than non-smokers who live in rural areas.

Could the cause of breast cancer be staring us in the face?

ASSOCIATION AND CAUSE

Studies are constantly being carried out to find out whether or not there is an association between diet and cancer, pollution and cancer and so on. However, finding an association between diet and cancer does not prove that diet causes cancer.

Some of the greatest advances in medicine were by those who observed their patients, took note of everything that was happening around them, came up with an idea, and carried out tests to see if they were correct.

In the 19th century, most woman delivered their babies at home, but many, mainly the poor, gave birth in hospital, where many died from infection (known as puerperal fever) in far greater numbers than those who gave birth elsewhere. Women began to notice this, and rejected hospital care whenever possible. They had noticed an association between hospital deliveries and an increase in death rates. They had no idea what caused the increased number of deaths, but they already knew that they were less likely to die from childbirth if they had their baby at home. Doctors at the time assumed that it was inevitable that many women would die in childbirth, and so believed that such deaths could not be avoided.

Dr. Ignas Semmelweis (known as the "saviour of women") worked in the maternity hospital in Vienna. He was puzzled by the fact that far more women died in the ward nearest to the dissecting room than in another ward. The wards were identical, except that medical students were taught in the first one and midwives in the second. As midwives did not work in the dissecting room, Dr. Semmelweis thought that perhaps the medical students carried something on their hands from the dead bodies they had examined to the women they then examined during labour. Even though no-one knew anything about germs at the time (it was not even known that such things existed) he ordered all students to wash their hands before they examined each woman in the labour ward. The death rate dropped dramatically from about thirty women in every hundred to about one woman in a hundred.

Even with such an incredible drop in the death rate, his theory still wasn't accepted. As far as his superiors were concerned he was talking utter rubbish. Medical journals wrote that "it was time he stopped his nonsense about hand-washing." Despite the ridicule, Dr. Semmelweis continued the practice, and death rates in the hospital where he worked remained low. His advice was ignored in other hospitals, and women there died in their thousands. It was only after his death, decades later, that his theory was accepted by medical science.

The tests carried out by Dr. Semmelweis did not put anyone's life at risk, nor did he find the cause of the "fever" which killed so many women. However, the result of his theory saved thousands of lives.

Trials in the past were not always carried out with such considera-tion for patients. The tests carried out by scientists which eventu-ally led to the discovery of the smallpox vaccine is one such case.

Dr. Edward Jenner noticed that milkmaids who had suffered from cow-pox, a fairly harmless disease, didn't get smallpox. He decid-ed to find out what would happen if he infected a person with cow-pox, and then infected that same person with smallpox, a disease which was always very serious and frequently caused death. He carried out this procedure on a young healthy boy who fortunately lived to tell the tale. Further tests were carried out on others with the same success.

Nowadays, no one in their right mind would approve of this kind of human experimentation to obtain scientific evidence. Consequently, it can sometimes be almost impossible to get ade-quate proof of cause and effect.

There is no absolute evidence to show that the eating of affected beef causes the human variant of mad cow disease (CJD). It is most unlikely that a few hundred people will volunteer to eat beef which has been proven to be infected with BSE to see whether or not they will die. In the absence of such direct evidence, surveys on the association between CJD in humans, and the mere likelihood of their being infected with the disease by eating infected beef, will have to continue.

If ongoing trials were to demonstrate that the disease was most common in those who had eaten a lot of beef during the time when some of the beef contained BSE, it would be accepted as showing some evidence. So, time will pass, and surveys will be carried out.

Post mortems will be carried out on all people who die of CJD, and attempts will be made to establish links between their disease and their consumption of potentially infected beef. Then, if it is shown that only those who have eaten beef go on to get CJD, there will be evidence to show that there is a strong association between the consumption of beef and CJD in humans. It will still not prove that the illness was caused by the meat, as the meat might not have been infected.

It is even more complicated when it comes to breast cancer, as there is no particular factor associated with the disease, but many different ones. However, the evidence linking breast cancer with the consumption of oestrogens is far greater than the evidence which links mad cow disease with CJD in humans.

Until the principal causes of breast cancer have been established, which could take decades, women will have to make their own decisions with regard to what measures they will take to avoid getting breast cancer.

BREAST DISEASE

The word "tumour", especially associated with the breast, fills most women with dread. Even if they are told it is a benign tumour, some women don't understand the word "benign", while others don't even hear the word being mentioned because of their state of anxiety.

To many, the word "tumour" means "cancer." Even though their doctor may have given them good news, the unfortunate women hear the worst, and go through the same ordeal that they would have gone through had they been told that they had cancer.

* The word "tumour" means "lump".

* The word "benign" means "harmless".

* A benign tumour is a harmless lump (more on that later).

* A malignant tumour is cancer.

* Ninety per cent of all lumps examined are harmless.

What is a Harmless Lump?

A harmless lump is caused by the abnormal division of normal cells which are contained inside a covering of skin. These cells continue to look like the cells outside the lump both in size and shape. Cells inside a harmless lump do not travel around the body.

What is a Cancerous Lump?

A cancerous lump is caused by the uncontrolled division of abnormal cells which form a lump inside a covering of skin. These cells are different in size and shape from the normal cells and can be different in size and shape from each other. Cancer can take from ten to twenty years to become noticable. Some cancer cells grow slowly and others quite quickly. Cancer cells can travel to other parts of the body.

What is Breast Disease?

When women hear the words "breast disease" they immediately think of breast cancer. The term "breast disease" covers other problems such as cysts, pain, lumps, mastitis, discharge, abscesses and so on which, after examination, have been found to be "harmless". In other words they are medical problems which are not cancerous.

Normally cells in our bodies multiply in an organised way. However, sometimes something happens to a cell in the breast which sends it berserk and it starts multiplying like mad. After a while, there are so many extra abnormal cells in one place that they form a small lump. This is known as a "primary cancer." The cancer cells are all confined inside the lump. These cells just stay where they are, sometimes for years, but eventually some of them decide they have had enough. They escape, get into the blood stream, and go wandering off to set up camp somewhere else. When they settle in another organ, these delinquent cells continue their lawless behaviour, reproduce without control and form a second lump.

This second lump is a "secondary cancer" or "metastasis", which is the medical word used to confuse us.

Some cancer cells, which multiply until they have formed a lump, are quite happy to stay in one place, and do not go wandering about the body for years on end. Many women will have died of old age before this happens.

As we do not yet know which cells will stay in one place and which will go wandering into the blood stream, you can understand why it is necessary to have a lump removed while the cancer cells are still inside. Once they get outside the lump they are more difficult to control.

Cancer cells aren't happy just setting up camp in your body, they need food to keep multiplying. In most cases their food is oestrogen.

Once a lump is removed with all the cells still inside, patients are often given a drug called Tamoxifen. This is an anti-oestrogen drug, which stops our own natural oestrogens from having their normal effects on our bodies. It prevents any cancer cells which might still be wandering about from getting enough oestrogen to continue multiplying. In a way these cells are starved to death.

The big question is *why* do cells become abnormal and start to multiply uncontrollably? It is not known why cells change, but it is now known that *oestrogens* cause cancer cells to multiply. Could it be that normal cells which get too much oestrogen become abnormal and then continue to divide because of the increased levels of this hormone? Some scientists believe that we all have cancer cells, and that these are kept in check naturally by the body. It is only when things go wrong in some way that the cancer cells multiply.

It has only recently been discovered that chemicals which have an oestrogenic effect can cause cancer cells to multiply. As oestrogens cause cancer cells to multiply, it would seem rational to find out if oestrogen added to normal cells caused them to become cancerous. This is such a simple idea that tests to prove it have probably been carried out umpteen times, but for the life of me I cannot find any mention of such tests in any of the numerous text books or clinical papers I have read over the years.

Much of what is known about breast cancer points to oestrogens as being a likely cause. This may be due to our own production of the hormone. For example, it is believed that increased consumption of protein and fat (mainly animal fat), and a decrease of fibre in our diet causes changes in the gut, so that oestrogens which would otherwise be excreted from the body are reabsorbed. This leads to high oestrogen levels in our body. Of course, taking the pill or HRT would also lead to higher oestrogen levels in our bodies, yet we are continually told that they are safe to use, and, in the case of HRT, we are informed that they are positively good for us.

Why should so many women have something wrong with their own hormones which results in cancer? Judging by the cause of other forms of cancer in the past, it seems likely that the increase in breast cancer is more likely to be due to external factors.

THE INTRODUCTION OF HORMONES

If we are to get a better understanding of breast disease, we must consider the changes in medical practice, lifestyles and industrial developments which have taken place over the past forty years.

The biggest thing that happened to women during this time was the development of the contraceptive Pill.

Until the 20th century, governments were mainly interested in increasing family size, and the idea of limiting the number of children in a family never entered their heads.

Early in the 19th century, groups were formed to encourage discussion on ways of preventing conception within marriage, such as sexual abstinence. They made little progress, due to continual attacks by the medical profession and the church. Laws were then passed against the "vice of contraception", which would have included using "the safe period", had they known anything about it at the time, which of course they did not. Sexual intercourse between single consenting adults was then a crime, and remains so in some American states, even though these laws are now ignored.

In 1916, two sisters opened a contraception advice clinic and were therefore arrested. However, the court's findings enabled doctors to give contraceptive advice "for prevention or cure of any disease". Married couples still could not legally limit the size of their family by any means whatsoever, even if their lives and that of their children were a total misery as a result of poverty. Not surprisingly, the American movement grew.

In 1927, a birth-control investigation committee was set up in London and, after much research, a substance which kills sperm (spermicide) was produced for use by an "approved list" of people, mainly married women in medical need.

The first birth control pill was approved in the USA in the 1960s after only short-term testing on small numbers of women. Within ten years of its discovery, seven million women were taking the drug, as it was very effective and easy to use.

This early Pill contained very high levels of oestrogen (150mcg), which, at the time, was believed to be totally safe to use, but in fact caused serious side-effects and deaths in women.

Because of the difficulties in measuring female hormone levels, the dose was based on experiments which were only interested in the amount required to prevent conception, and which could still be tolerated by women. In 1969, the British Committee on the Safety of Drugs recommended that all doctors prescribe the lower dose oestrogen pills which had come on the market, as there was evidence to show that oestrogens increased the risk of blood clots. Since then, the amount of oestrogen in the Pill has been reduced regularly to the current level of between 30mcg and 50mcg.

There are two main types of Pill. The *combined Pill*, which contains oestrogen and progesterone, and the *progesterone only Pill*, also known as the mini pill. It has now been established that even these lower dose Pills increase the risk of blood clots in users.

It has been agreed for some time that there is only a small risk of breast cancer associated with the use of the Pill. But, as millions of women use the Pill, this small risk affects huge numbers of women. As time passes, the results of more recent surveys show higher risks than those published some time ago. The result of just one recent survey shows that young women who take the Pill for four or more years before their first pregnancy are twice as likely to get breast cancer before they reach the menopause than women who do not take it

We continue to be told that pregnancy is more dangerous than taking the Pill.

Is this really true to-day?

It must be remembered that, to prevent one pregnancy which lasts nine months, the Pill may have to be taken for years. It is accepted, even by the drug companies, that 6.6 women in one hundred thousand will die from thrombosis (a clot) due to taking the newer low-dose Pill, and that 3.3 women in one hundred thousand will die of the same disease among those who take the higher dose Pill.

The death rate in this country due to pregnancy is 3.2 per 100,000, which is less than the number of deaths due to taking the "safer" Pill.

It is known that more women who take the Pill die of cancer than those who have never taken it. But, as it has not yet been proven that these deaths were directly due to taking the Pill, the number of deaths due to cancer from taking it is not yet known. However, even if we only take deaths due to thromboses into account, we can see that pregnancy is safer than taking the Pill.

However, if those now taking the Pill had to use other forms of contraception, there could be "accidents," leading to more pregnancies. On the other hand, its use is not 100% reliable, either as one can forget to take it on a particular day, or because certain drugs interfere with its effectiveness.

Some of the side-effects of the Pill are:

High blood pressure.

Depression.

Gall-bladder disease.*

Weight-gain.

Thrombosis (the formation of a clot).

Stroke.

Nausea.

Headache.

Mastalgia.

Loss of sexual desire.

An increased risk of breast cancer.

The Pill interferes with women to such an extent that it causes them to be infertile while they take it. Just because this is the intention does not mean it is a safe form of contraception.

(*During the 1960s, gall-bladder disease was extremely rare and was only found mainly in women. One way of remembering who suffered from the problem (for exam purposes) was to think of the three "Fs": Female, Fat and Forty. Over the years, there has been a large increase in the number of women, and a huge increase in the number of men suffering from this disease. As men do not take the Pill or HRT, one must wonder whether or not it may be due to the increased consumption of hormones in their diet, particularly those found in meat.)

HRT

When HRT came into general use 30 years ago it was considered to be a perfectly safe form of treatment, as it contained oestrogen which was "just a hormone women produced naturally." It was later discovered that this "perfectly safe" use of oestrogen greatly increased the risk of cancer of the womb. After this discovery, it was recommended that progesterone be added to the treatment to reduce this risk.

Some women sail through the menopause without any bother, some have mild problems, while others have more severe ones. These problems are caused by changing levels of oestrogens in the body. Why some women have such problems and others do not is unknown.

HRT reduces hot flushes, night sweats and mood changes. There is also evidence which shows that it can reduce the loss of bone strength (osteoporosis), which would otherwise cause bones to break easily. Many studies now show an increased risk of breast cancer in women who take HRT for more than five years, and only time will tell whether women who take HRT for a shorter time are also at risk.

Many pelvic diseases such as fibroids often naturally regress after the menopause, but women are now being encouraged to undergo HRT, which can reactivate these diseases. This is so that they can have the benefits of HRT, such as a reduction of the risk of heart disease and stroke. But oestrogen alone increases the risk of womb cancer, and the addition of progesterone cancels out the possible reduction in heart disease. This advice is even given to women who have no menopausal problems, even though the long-term effects of HRT are not yet known. Women on this therapy are the first generation to try out the treatment for long periods, and are therefore part of a very large clinical trial.

The menopause is not a disease. It is a natural part of women's lives, during which some may need treatment to help with hot flushes or night sweats. These can be treated with non-hormonal drugs or natural remedies.

Puberty is also a time of change in our lives, but teenagers with acne who go to their doctor do not expect to be put on hormones to "get them through puberty." They want medication to clear up their spots. Will hormonal treatment for puberty be the next step in the medicalisation of our lives?

Meat

Another change which occurred about 40 years ago was the introduction into the food chain of hormones, including oestrogen. Testosterone, progesterone, diethylstilbestrol, dienestrol and oestradiol were given to livestock in various combinations as growth promoters.

Twenty years later, one of these hormones, diethylstilbestrol, known as DES, was banned when it was discovered that children of women who took the drug got cancer of the vagina as a consequence.

Before that time, vaginal cancer was one of the rarest forms of cancer, and was almost unheard of in women under 50 years of age. DES is also associated with an increased risk of breast cancer in women who were given the hormone during pregnancy.

Women around the world took this hormone to prevent miscarriage but it is now known that it can in fact cause miscarriage. During the 1970s, DES was considered the drug of choice for many problems as it was cheap and could be taken by mouth.

Some of the uses of DES were:

* To control hot flushes during the menopause.

* To suppress the secretion of breast milk after childbirth.

* To treat some cases of breast cancer.

* To treat delayed puberty in teenage girls.

It must also be pointed out that most women were eating meat containing DES for about twenty years, whether pregnant or not, and the effects of this are still unknown.

The remaining growth-promoting hormones continued to be used until they were banned by the EU in 1981. They were banned in Ireland in 1988.

Scientific evidence has shown that there is an increased risk of breast cancer in women who eat a high-fat diet (mainly animal fat). It seems to be ignored that the cause may not be the fat, but rather the assortment of hormones (including oestrogen) in the fat which is delivered through livestock to our dinner tables.

The introduction of hormones into the food chain may yet prove to have been one of the worst disasters of our time.

CHEMICALS

The widespread use of chemicals also took place during the last 40 years, and now poses a threat to all living creatures. These chemicals are in the air, rivers, lakes and sea. They are in the soil and, worst of all, they are sprayed on the food we eat.

Many chemicals remain in the environment and accumulate over the years. The use of DDT, which was reduced to a large extent in the 1970s, has been found in agricultural soil at rates of up to 100 lbs per acre, and is still used in certain circumstances today.

Many birds became almost extinct due to eating DDT-treated seeds. Some of these birds may have died from poisoning, but the huge decline in their numbers was mainly due to reproductive failure.

It is now known that DDT acts like a weak form of oestrogen and can damage the hormonal system. Women who have high levels of DDT in their blood have four times the risk of getting breast cancer than women with no DDT.

Over the years, hundreds of new chemicals have been produced and are in use all over the world.

Testicular cancer has trebled, and undescended testis has doubled in Britain and America in the past thirty years. Many men who were exposed to the oestrogen DES while in the womb have been found to have low sperm counts. However, many men who were not exposed to DES while in the womb also have low sperm counts, and it is now believed that this may be due to the effect of chemicals in food which have an oestrogenic effect.

These are not chemically made oestrogens, but are other chemicals which have the same effect on the body as oestrogens. These chemicals are called "Oestrogenics."

If substances found in chemicals have an oestrogenic effect on males, must they not also have an oestrogenic effect on females? And if these chemicals have such disastrous effects on humans, then surely oestrogens in meat must also have disastrous effects on everyone?

Large-scale studies are being carried out to examine the oestrogenic effect of chemicals on humans. However, there is almost no research being carried out on the effects of oestrogens in meat and milk, even though these hormones are still legally used in livestock in America and in other countries. Even though hormones have been banned in the EU, enforcement of these regulations has proved to be almost impossible.

During the past 40 years or so we have been bombarded with hormones, especially oestrogens and oestrogen-like substances which are now believed to have drastic consequences on humans as well as on animals.

If it is accepted that the residues of oestrogens in meat can have such dire consequences when fed to people in general, why should we believe that the same hormone in tablet form is good for women?

DRUG TESTING

Numerous tests are performed on new drugs before they can be given to humans. Even then, large numbers of people must volunteer to take part in controlled trials before medicines are put on the market. In these trials, neither the patients nor the observers know who is getting the drug or who is getting the "dummy" pills. Then, if it is found that the patients on the drug have done better without serious side-effects than those on the dummy pill, there is evidence of the drug's value. If the new product is found to cause serious side-effects it cannot be used.

However, disasters do still occur, especially when side-effects do not show up for months or even years after the drug has been taken. Examples of this were the thalidomide and DES disasters.

When it comes to giving millions of people drugs in their food, no such tests are carried out. It is not until after disasters occur that anything is done about it. When it comes to hormones in meat (and now milk), millions of people are the unknowing guinea-pigs.

Studies which attempt to measure the effect of added oestrogens have shown that women who take them in the Pill over a number of years have only a slightly increased chance of developing cancer than women who have not been on the pill at all. Is this true?

The problem with most existing studies is that they have only taken into consideration those oestrogens which are administered by doctors. They have totally failed to acknowledge the effect of extra oestrogens in meat and other foods which are being eaten by women. This is not how properly conducted trials should be carried out.

As we have seen, drug trials must compare the effects of a drug on patients who are taking it against those who have not taken the drug in any form. This is not what is being done when looking at the effects of the Pill and HRT on women. If it were, they would give different results. What we have with regard to the Pill and HRT is the legalised selling of drugs which have never been properly tested.

The only way to have conducted these tests would have been to compare vast numbers of vegetarian women on the Pill with vegetarian women who had never taken the Pill or HRT.

Even organic meat contains natural oestrogens, so we must then ask whether the increased consumption of meat, even without added hormones, during the past forty years could have caused the increase in cancers.

There is no scientific answer to this but even if the answer was "yes", then the addition of even more hormones could only make matters worse.

In the early 1980s, the scientific group of the Commission of the European Communities found no reason to conclude that the use of oestradiol-17, testosterone and progesterone (hormones including oestrogens), used as growth promoters in animals for human consumption should be banned, because they found no evidence to show that their use was harmful to the consumer. In other words, as far as the experts were concerned, these hormones were perfectly safe. Yet subsequently these substances were banned by the EU.

They were hardly banned for the good of the animals, as they were being prepared for slaughter. Nor could they have been banned for the sake of the meat industry, as hormones increase weight in animals at little cost to farmers, thereby giving more income to all involved. So one can only assume that during the thirty-plus years while we were happily eating our hormone-laced meat, someone discovered that these hormones were not as safe as they thought. Indeed, they were causing so much harm to the meat trade, never mind the unfortunate consumer, that they would have to be banned, even though such a step would bring about a huge drop in profits in the meat market throughout the entire EU.

In some EU countries hormone-trafficking is now the most profitable crime after drug-dealing. One must ask: Where are all these hormones going?

Milk

Another fairly recent legal use of vast quantities of hormones has been that of the hormone known as BST (oestrogen) in dairy cattle. By giving the animals this drug, milk production is increased by 10%. However, trials have shown that 50% of these animals who have been given this hormone get mastitis (an infection of the udder).

To prevent pus from getting into the milk, these animals have to be treated with antibiotics. Even though there is the cost of BST to each cow, and the cost of antibiotics to 50% of the animals to produce 10% more milk, it must be profitable, as this hormone-produced milk is now on sale in America and other non-EU countries. Mind you, the fact that the milk is produced by injecting the animals with hormones and antibiotics is *not* printed on the containers. If there are "trials" being carried out in other countries, including those in the EU, we, the consumers, are unlikely to know about them. The fact that the milk was produced from cows who had been treated with hormones and antibiotics would be a well-kept secret.

It is also worrying to realise that 50% of cows treated with the hormone BST get mastitis. If there are traces of BST in the milk we drink, is it not possible that humans are also likely to suffer from the ingestion of this hormone?

Once again there have been no long-term studies to determine the effects of BST on humans, only on cows.

It has now been accepted by medical experts that changing the hormonal balance of women encourages cancer growth. As anti-oestrogen drugs are used in the treatment of breast cancer, it is reasonable to assume that hormones taken in food may be an underlying cause of the disease.

Warnings

Many illnesses are dose-related. For example, a person who smokes 50 cigarettes a day is far more likely to die from lung cancer than someone who smokes five cigarettes a day. It also takes years for lung cancer to develop, but there are usually early warning signs, such as a "smokers cough", before cancer is diagnosed.

When it comes to breast cancer and other female-type cancers, there are no noticeable warning signs before cancer is diagnosed. Or are there?

With regard to breast lumps, most women go to their doctor as soon as possible. After the lump has been examined, women are told whether or not it is cancer. When it is *not* cancer, they are told they are fine, and there are no further investigations.

When it comes to severe breast pain, most women are told what it is *not* due to. They are not told why they have the pain, and, in most cases, are not given any treatment. One would imagine that women cannot tell the difference between pain and discomfort.

There are not many people who would continue going to a dentist who only told them what their toothache was *not* due to. These patients would want something done about the pain, and they would certainly not put up with being told that their pain was normal.

*

Imagine the following scenario:

Patient: *I'm in agony with a toothache.*
Dentist: *Sit down there and let me have a look. Open wide. PAUSE. There's absolutely nothing to worry about, it's not cancer.*
Patient: *But I've an awful toothache.*
Dentist: *That's quite normal...perfectly normal.*
Patient: *But...*
Dentist: *I've examined your entire mouth and there isn't a sign of cancer. You mustn't worry, you're fine.*

If people went to such dentists, they would think the dentists were mad, but we accept this kind of care when it comes to breast pain, or "harmless" lumps.

Fortunately things are slowly changing, and a small number of women is being given treatment for breast pain. One of the drugs used is Tamoxifen (anti-oestrogen), which has been shown in clinical trials to have beneficial effects, thus proving that the condition may be caused by oestrogens. But what about women who have breast pain and are not on oestrogen either in the form of the Pill or HRT? It seems highly likely that oestrogens in meat and/or milk may play a role in the production of many such diseases in women.

* Oestrogens in the Pill and HRT can cause breast pain.

72

* Breast pain is due to increased oestrogen in the body.

* Many breast cancers are also caused by increased oestrogen levels.

* It seems likely that breast pain and "harmless" breast lumps may be a warning sign or a pre-cancerous condition.

Scientific surveys show that there is an association between breast pain and breast cancer, but there is no proof that breast pain or a harmless lump is a pre-cancerous condition. What this also means is that there is no proof that these problems are *not* pre-cancerous conditions.

SIGNS AND SYMPTOMS

The number of women suffering from pelvic disease such as fibroids and endometriosis is increasing every year. A common complaint among women with pelvic disease is lower abdominal pain. According to research, these conditions are in some way related to oestrogens in our bodies, and there is no known cause for these diseases. All treatments interfere with women's natural hormones, and can cause menopausal, or "male type" symptoms, which, in some cases, are irreversible.

The reason I mention pelvic conditions is that while eating ordinary chicken I also had lower abdominal pain (as well as the breast pain). A urine test showed that there was no infection. After months of "on and off" pain, I began to notice that it happened about once a month and lasted for about a week. When I finally gave up eating all poultry, both the mastalgia and the lower abdominal pain were completely cured.

I have no idea whether this lower abdominal pain had anything to do with fibroids or endometriosis, as no diagnosis was made. However, I wonder whether this type of pain could be an early sign of pelvic disease due to oestrogens in our diet, especially in meat.

In the 1960s and 1970s, scientists were only just beginning to find ways of measuring women's oestrogen levels. Experiments had been carried out by injecting women with oestrogens, and it was found that 10% of the injected oestrogen was excreted in the urine. With this knowledge, they could work out the natural levels of oestrogen. By examining the urine of women, they found that, on average, women passed 1mg of oestrogen each cycle. Therefore the amount produced by the body would be 10mg each cycle.

Just because women pass 1mg of oestrogen in their urine does not mean that this amount was naturally produced, as at the time of these tests women were eating oestrogen-laced meat daily.

All that was learned from these experiments was the average amount of oestrogen found in the urine of women. It does not give the normal oestrogen levels naturally produced by women. Now that we live in a sea of oestrogens, it will be difficult (but not impossible) to establish what are the normal levels of oestrogens in women.

As oestrogens play such an important role in cancer cell growth, we need facts concerning the results of scientific tests for hormones carried out on animals for human consumption, especially with regard to poultry. We also need independent, up-to-date information on the effects of the Pill and HRT. We need to be told the truth, so that we can make decisions for ourselves, decisions which may prevent disease.

In America, where hormones, including oestrogens, are legally used as growth promoters in livestock, where meat consumption is high and breast cancer rates are amongst the highest in the world, young healthy women who have a close relative with breast cancer have been put on anti-oestrogen drugs. This trial is being carried out in the hope that such treatment will prevent these women from getting breast cancer later in life.

This may seem reasonable, as many breast cancers need oestrogens to grow. However, to interfere with women's natural hormone levels while feeding them meat and milk laced with hormones makes no sense whatsoever.

It does not take a genius to work out that it would make far more sense to stop feeding women hormones to see if it will prevent them getting cancer later on, than to first increase their hormone levels by giving them added hormones in their food, and then to decrease those levels with drugs.

Of course, sense doesn't come into this, what we are looking at is greed. By changing women's very being, all those in the meat and milk trade can continue to profit by being legally permitted to use hormones as growth promoters, and to increase milk yields. The profit to be made by drug companies is huge.

As we have seen, most cancers are the result of environmental factors affecting people. As far as the medical world is concerned, the whole problem with women is that they are women. It is we who are flawed - we produce oestrogens.

In their attempt to treat problems probably due to external causes, they alter our hormones - the very essence of femininity - instead of trying to find the true, external, cause of breast disease.

Over twenty billion dollars is spent on cancer research in America each year, mainly on expensive machines and drugs to diagnose and treat the disease, but only a tiny proportion of this money (about 2%) is spent on looking for the cause of cancer.

Until this cause is known, the only option open to women is fear, routine examination and experimental treatment.

My own experience and the results of the survey and clinical trial, together with other medical evidence, gives me reason to believe that oestrogens given to livestock, and subsequently eaten by us, have many adverse effects on women's health, and may even be the cause of many forms of breast disease.

Mastalgia and poultry consumption

Clancy. A.M.

Abstract

An epidemiological survey was carried out to determine whether mastalgia is associated with the consumption of meat or poultry, with the taking of hormones or with smoking.

Mastalgia was present in 21.8% of the 119 women surveyed. The results show a greater than four-fold increase of mastalgia in women who consume above average amounts of chicken [O.R. 4.60 95%CL < OR 1.67 < 12.88].

There was a weak association between the taking of the contraceptive pill (CP) and mastalgia.

It is suggested that hormones in poultry may be the factor in chicken which causes mastalgia.

Introduction

Many women suffer from some degree of breast pain, usually associated with tenderness for a few days prior to menstruation, but there seems to be little information on the prevalence of the more severe pain (mastalgia) in the community.

This study of women in an Irish town was conducted in an attempt to establish the prevalence of mastalgia, and to look at the possible association between the condition and hormones, smoking and dietary factors.

Method

A random survey of women was undertaken by the author who surveyed women in five selected areas in a town of 8,000 people. Using a systematic sampling method, one in every three houses was surveyed to obtain a sample of 25 in each area. Only women aged 30 or over were included in the survey.

The questionnaire includes 25 specific questions relating to meat and poultry consumption, the taking of the Pill, HRT, smoking and details of duration and degree of breast pain.

In establishing the types of meats eaten, distinction was made between organic and non-organic meat and poultry. Very few women were eating organic meat and poultry and, unless otherwise stated, "chicken" and "meat" in the text refers to non-organic produce. Women were categorised as being "Low, Mod, or High" consumers based on the average amounts consumed in meals and the number of such meals eaten weekly. In traditional cooking it was found that an adult portion of chicken was about 6oz and that of meat about 4oz. Where Eastern-style cooking was used, portions were approximately 50% less, and allowance was made for this when categorising women in respect of amount eaten.

Table 1. Categorisation of chicken & meat consumers.

Type of meat	Category		
	Low	Mod	High
Chicken	<1 meal/wk.	1 meal/wk.	>1 meal/wk.
Other Meat	<3 meal/wk.	3-4 meal/wk.	>4 meal/wk.
Standard meal:	*Chicken*	*6oz.*	
	Other Meat	*4oz.*	

Mastalgia was defined as severe, diffuse, bilateral breast pain, tender to the touch, most acute in the upper, outer quadrants and lasting a minimum of 4 days each month. Pain was categorised in the following manner:

	Degree of pain	Category
A	Normal levels of breast pain	No pain
B	Severe pain for 4-6 days	Moderate
C	Severe pain for 1 week or more	High

Results.

From a total sample of 125 women, 119 completed the question-naire. The mean age was 46.6 years and 63% were aged <50yrs. None of the six women who were either vegetarian or organic meat & poultry eaters suffered from mastalgia.

Seventeen women (14.3%) had undergone biopsy of the breast, one of whom was diagnosed malignant.

Twenty six women (21.8%) suffered from mastalgia and only one of these had received medical treatment for the condition.

39.5% had taken the Pill at some time, while 11% were on the Pill when surveyed. An association between taking the Pill and mastal-gia was demonstrated, Odds ratio: 1.74.

95% CL $0.66 < OR < 4.60$, but this was not statistically significant.

6% had taken HRT.

31% had smoked cigarettes, but there was no association between smoking and mastalgia.

There was a strong association between the amount of chicken eaten and the prevalence of mastalgia.

Table 2 demonstrates that while 40% of high chicken consumers suffered from mastalgia, only 11% of Low and 13.5% of Mod. chicken consumers suffered from the condition.

Table 2. Prevalence of mastalgia according to category of chicken consumption.

Amount chicken	Mastalgia +	-	Total
High	16	24	40
Low*	03	24	27
Mod	07	45	52
Total	26	93	119

Chi square = 11.68, DF = 2, P <0.001

*Vegetarians are within the definition of eating less than one meal of chicken/week and are therefore categorised as "Low".

Table 3 demonstrates the increased risk (OR 4.60) of mastalgia in women who eat "high" amounts of chicken.

Table 3. Odds of mastalgia in high chicken consumers.

High poultry	Mastalgia +	-	Total
+	16	24	40
-	10	69	79
Total	26	93	119

Odds ratio   4.60   95% CL 1.67 <OR <12.88

Relative risk   3.16   95% CL 1.58 < RR <6.32

Chi-Square   11.63   P<0.001

When the analysis is selected for age <50, the odds ratio increases from 4.6 to 5.5.

61% of women were categorised as "High" meat eaters, and no significant association was demonstrated between meat-eating and mastalgia.

Discussion

Many studies of mastalgia have been conducted on women attending breast clinics. Leinster et al[1] found that 69% of women attending for mammography had cyclical mastalgia. However such studies, having a highly selective sample, do not give a true indication of the prevalence of the disease in the community.

Increased prolactin stimulation, probably due to oestrogen dominance is a consistent finding in the aetiology of mastalgia.[2][3] The reduction of fat in the diet brings about striking relief in women with mastalgia.[4]

The possibility that oestrogens in meat may adversely effect humans has been considered. Perez Comas et al suggested the possibility that oestrogenic contamination of meat and poultry could explain the high incidence of abnormalities of sexual development in Puerto Rico.[5] Margaret Thorogood et al have shown a 40% reduction in mortality from cancer in vegetarian and fish eaters compared with meat eaters.[6]

Mastalgia should not be regarded as a simple matter of pain and discomfort. In a prospective study of 20,341 Seventh Day Adventist women carried out in California to determine the association between breast cancer and the use of HRT, it was demonstrated that women with prior benign breast disease showed a greater than two-fold risk (RR 2.80) of developing breast cancer than did the control group.[7]

Oestrogens and other hormones were introduced to livestock as growth promoters in the late 1950s and were used widely for almost thirty years. One of these hormones, DES, was banned in the 1970s as a result of abnormalities in children of DES treated women. The remaining hormones continued to be used widely despite being banned by the EEC in 1981. (81/602/EEC)

In September 1988, Ireland brought in regulations (SI No.218 of 1988) which prohibited the administration of Stilbene and its derivatives to any farm animal for human consumption. The use of substances having oestrogenic, androgenic or gestagenic effect was limited to the management of fertility related problems.

This legislation is to be welcomed. However, attempts to discover the results of routine screening of poultry for prohibited and controlled substances failed, as did attempts to have samples of poultry tested (PC DCC/MOH SEHB Feb. 1993).

It is a possibility that the increasing incidence of breast disease may be related more to the oestrogen content in animal fat rather than to the total quantity of fat consumed.

There is need to institute routine testing for hormones and oestrogen-like chemicals in poultry.

This study showed that mastalgia was quite common, having a prevalence of almost 22%, and just under 25% of these had one or more surgical biopsies.

It further demonstrated that there was an association between chicken consumption and mastalgia. Mastalgia was significantly more likely to occur in those who consumed "high" amounts of chicken as compared with those who ate "mod" or "low" amounts, and the association was greater in women under 50yrs. (OR 5.5)

None of the six women who were either vegetarian or organic meat eaters only suffered from mastalgia.

The study failed to demonstrate an association between consumption of meat (beef, pork or lamb) and mastalgia, but this may be related to the fact that most families ate meat at least three times weekly. Perhaps it would have been better to categorise most of the sample as being "high" meat eaters.

The study demonstrated an association between use of the contraceptive pill and mastalgia but this was not statistically significant.

This study demonstrates a very strong association between the consumption of higher than average amounts of chicken and the prevalence of mastalgia.

OR 4.6 95% CL 1.67 <OR <12.88.

It is essential that the findings in this epidemiological survey be further studied in clinical trials to establish whether there is a causal link between chicken consumption and mastalgia and if so which trace substances in chicken are the causative factors.

References

1. Leinster, S.J., Whitehouse, G.H., Walsh, P.V.: Cyclical Mastalgia: clinical and mammographic observations in a screened population. *Br J Surg 74: 220-2.*

2. Peters, F.: Multicenter study of gestrinone in cyclical breast pain. *Lancet 1992 339: 205-08.*

3. Peters, F., Schuth, W., Scheurich, B., Breckwoldt, M.: Serum prolactin levels in patients with fibrocystic breast disease. *Obstet Gynecol 1984; 64: 381-85.*

4. Boyd, N.F., Shannon, P., Kriukov, V., et al.: Effect of a low fat, high carbohydrate diet on symptoms of cyclical mastopathy. *Lancet 1988 1. 128-32.*

5. Perez-Comas, A., Saenz de Rodriquez, C.A., Sanchez Lugo, F.: Anomalias de Desarrollo Sexual en Puerto Rico. Estando de Situacion. *Bol Assoc. Med PR 1991. 83: 306-09.*

6. Thorogood, M., et al.: Risk of death from cancer and ischaemic heart disease in meat and non-meat eaters. *BMJ 1994. 308 1667-1669.*

7. Mills, P.K., Beeson, W.L., Phillips, R.L., Fraser, G.E.: Prospective study of exogenous hormone use and breast cancer in Seventh-day Adventists. *Cancer. 1989 64: 591-7.*

Clinical Trial on Women with Severe, Bilateral, Cyclical Mastalgia.

Clancy AM.

While a population survey on cyclical mastalgia was being conducted, nine women with severe mastalgia were randomly selected to take part in a clinical trial in April 1993. Only women with severe mastalgia who were at least 30 years old, were not taking hormone replacement therapy (HRT) or the contraceptive pill (the Pill), were included in the trial.

Severe mastalgia was defined as severe, bilateral breast pain for a minimum duration of seven days in each cycle.

All nine women had suffered from this condition for at least one year, and all had been recorded as being "mod" or "high" consumers of chicken

Moderate chicken consumption - 1 chicken meal per week.(approx. 6oz chicken)

High chicken consumption - 2 or more chicken meals/wk (12oz or more chicken)

*

The women were simply asked to eliminate all poultry from their diet and were informed that they would be interviewed again in six weeks time. No indication was given that this alteration in diet might have any effect on their level of breast pain. The general belief among the women was that "too much red meat was bad and chicken was good". No comment was made about this view.

On interview at six weeks all nine women claimed that they had refrained from eating chicken.

One woman detected no change in the level of breast pain while eight women said that they had become totally free of pain approximately two to three weeks after eliminating chicken from their diet and had remained pain-free.

It was then decided to challenge the pain-free women by getting them to revert to their original diet which included at least one meal of chicken (6oz min.) per week.

Four of the women, AM, BB, MB & AB agreed to resume eating chicken again while the other four women refused.

Of the four who agreed to revert to their chicken containing diet, three did so, AM, BB, & MB, and in all three women severe breast pain recurred within two to three weeks.

AM continued eating chicken for three months and then, because of pain, reduced her intake of chicken from 18oz per week to 6oz per week. At this moderate level of chicken intake she once again became pain-free and remained so (Feb.94.)

BB included chicken in her diet (12oz per week) for six weeks, but then felt compelled by pain to eliminate it once more. She again became pain-free and then decided to re-introduce a very small amount (3oz) of chicken once every three weeks. She has remained pain-free on this low intake (Feb.94).

MB did not initially revert to her pre-trial diet of 6oz of chicken per week, but decided to try eating 3oz of chicken weekly. However, after two weeks on this low chicken diet, her breast pain was so severe that she was once more forced to eliminate chicken from her diet. She again became pain-free and remains so (Feb 94).

AB did not revert to her pre-trial diet of 12oz of chicken weekly, but decided to opt for a chicken intake of 3oz per week. On this low chicken intake her breast pain did not recur and she remains pain-free to date (Feb 94).

Of the four women who refused to participate in the second stage of the trial, two have not eaten any chicken and have remained pain-free to date (Feb 94).

The other two women had chicken on two occasions and their breast pain returned each time. Both have reverted to a totally chicken-free diet and were pain-free for at least two months when checked in Feb 94.

Summary

Eight out of nine women suffering from severe, bilateral mastalgia of long duration became pain-free when placed on a chicken-free diet. They were followed up for a period of ten months and all were able to eliminate their symptoms by remaining on a low chicken diet or a chicken-free diet.

Publications also from On Stream,
available in bookstores or by mail-order:

Suicide The Irish Experience
Seán Spellissy **£6.99**

Tackling Men's Health, a guide to men's health & fitness.
Dr. John O'Riordan **£4.99**

French Country Roads, a wine-lover's guide to France *John D.O'Connell* **£6.99**

Tom Doorley Uncorked! Wine guide for purchasing in Ireland *Tom Doorley* **£5.99**

Developing On-Farm Research- the broad picture
Nora McNamara Stephen Morse **£9.99**

The Merchants of Ennis
Seán Spellissy **£12.99**

Memories of Macroom
James Kelleher **£4.99**

Cobh Now & Then
Joe Wilson **£6.50**

The Man from the Railway
James P. McNally **£4.99**

Pit Pony - Cavallo di miniera
Gerardo Vacana/Paolo Tullio **£7.50**

You May Talk Now!
Mary Phil Drennan **£4.99**

For mail-order/delivery send cheque/postal order for cost of the book plus £1.00 to:

Mail Order Dept. On Stream Publications Ltd. Cloghroe, Blarney, Co.Cork, Ireland.
Enquiries: Tel/fax + 353 21 385798. Email:onstream@indigo.ie